Adult Coloring Book 2

best adult stress relief coloring books for mindfulness and relaxation

MAGGIE DREAM

Introduction

Book Coloring - an excellent source of inspiration. While painting you may appear unusual ideas. If you are tired of the routine and want to do something nice, buy a coloring book and expand your creativity. Because of this you can do better at work.

Coloring Books for adults created in order to make you forget about all the current problems, and just relaxed.

Coloring beautiful picture, you forget about everything. At such moments, you become an artist and no work, no relationships do not disturb you.

Coloring Books for adults show you the beauty of the surrounding world. You forget about the gray gloomy everyday life, adding to your life more bright colors.

It was this book very quickly lead you into a good state of mind !!!

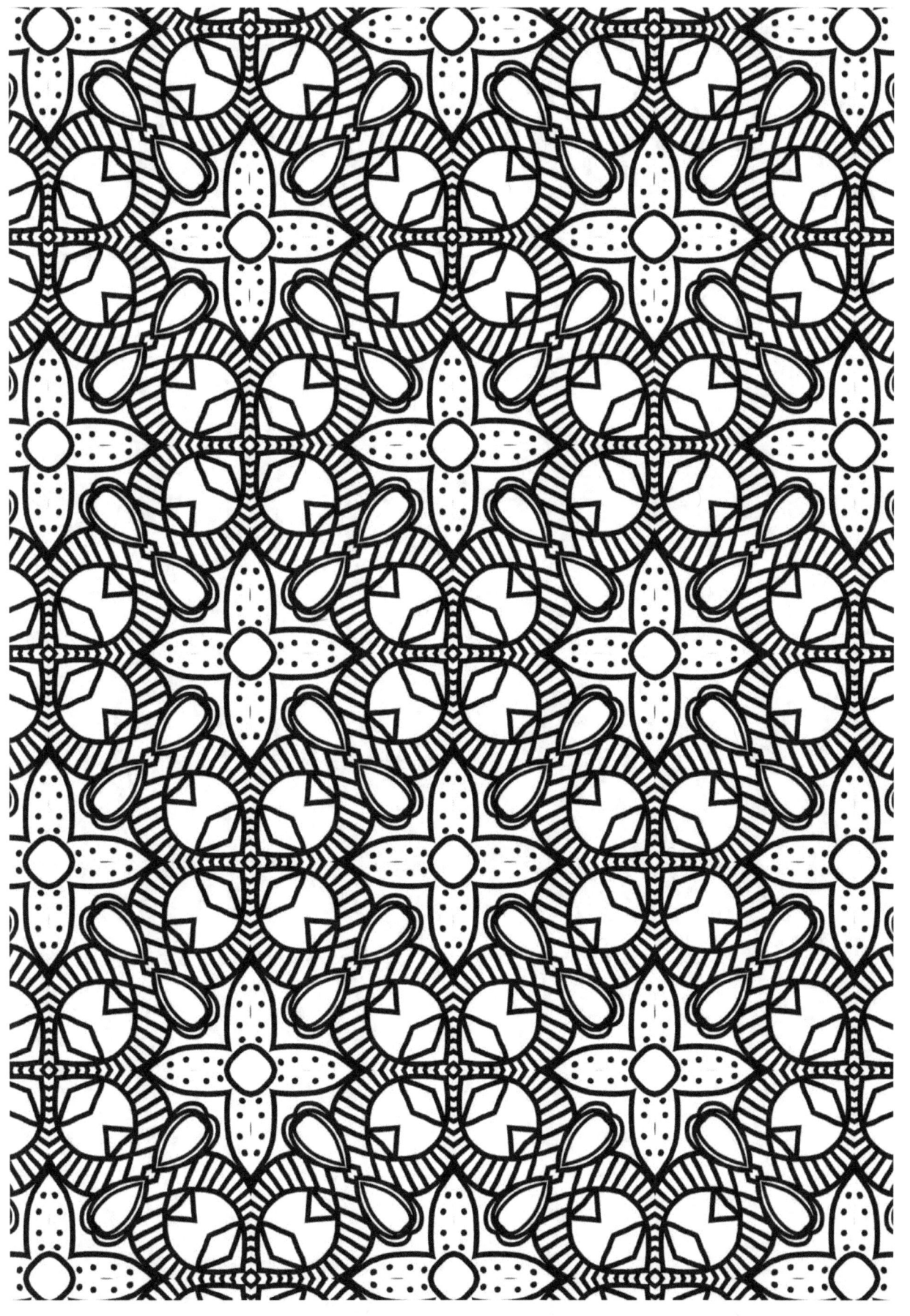

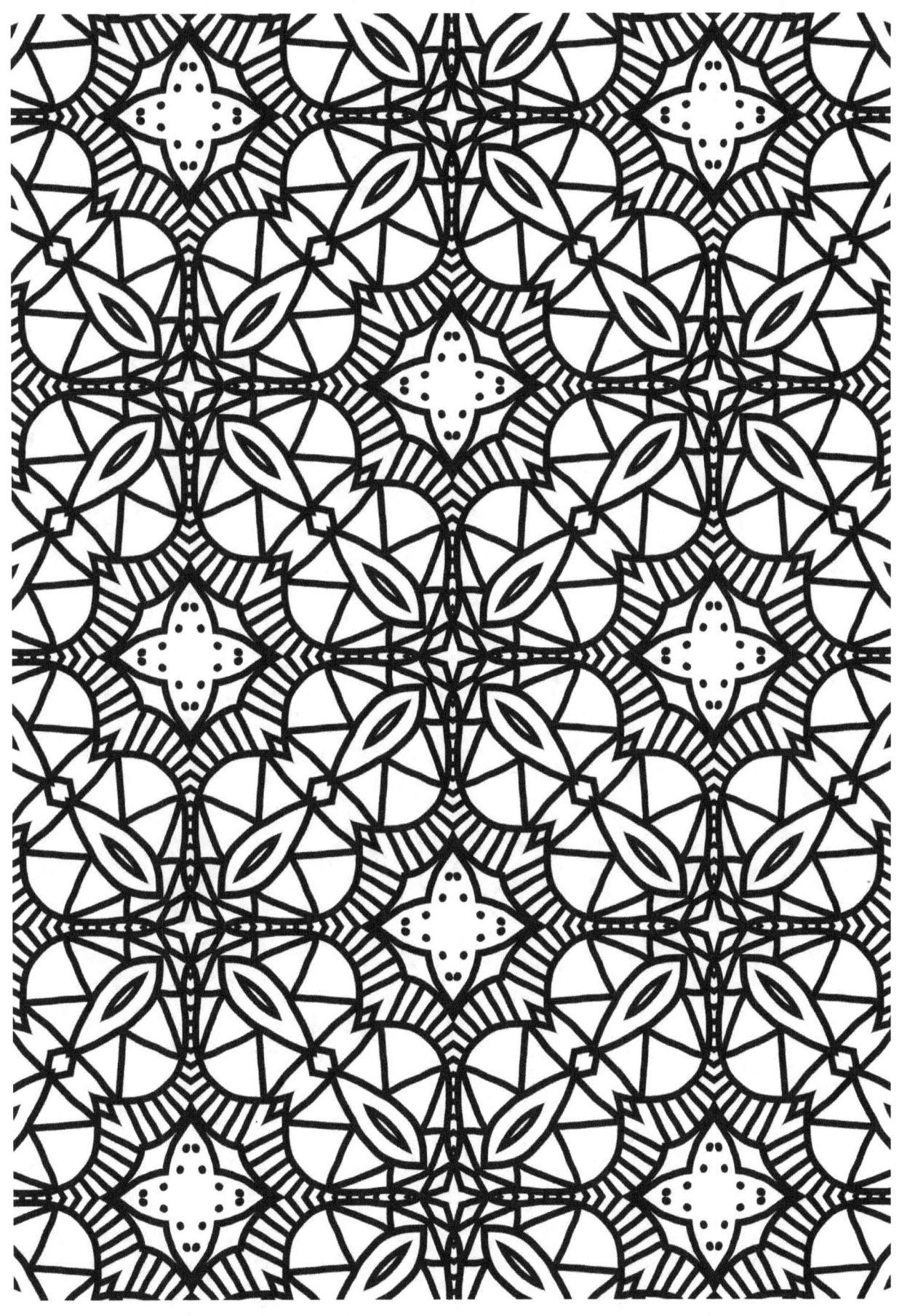

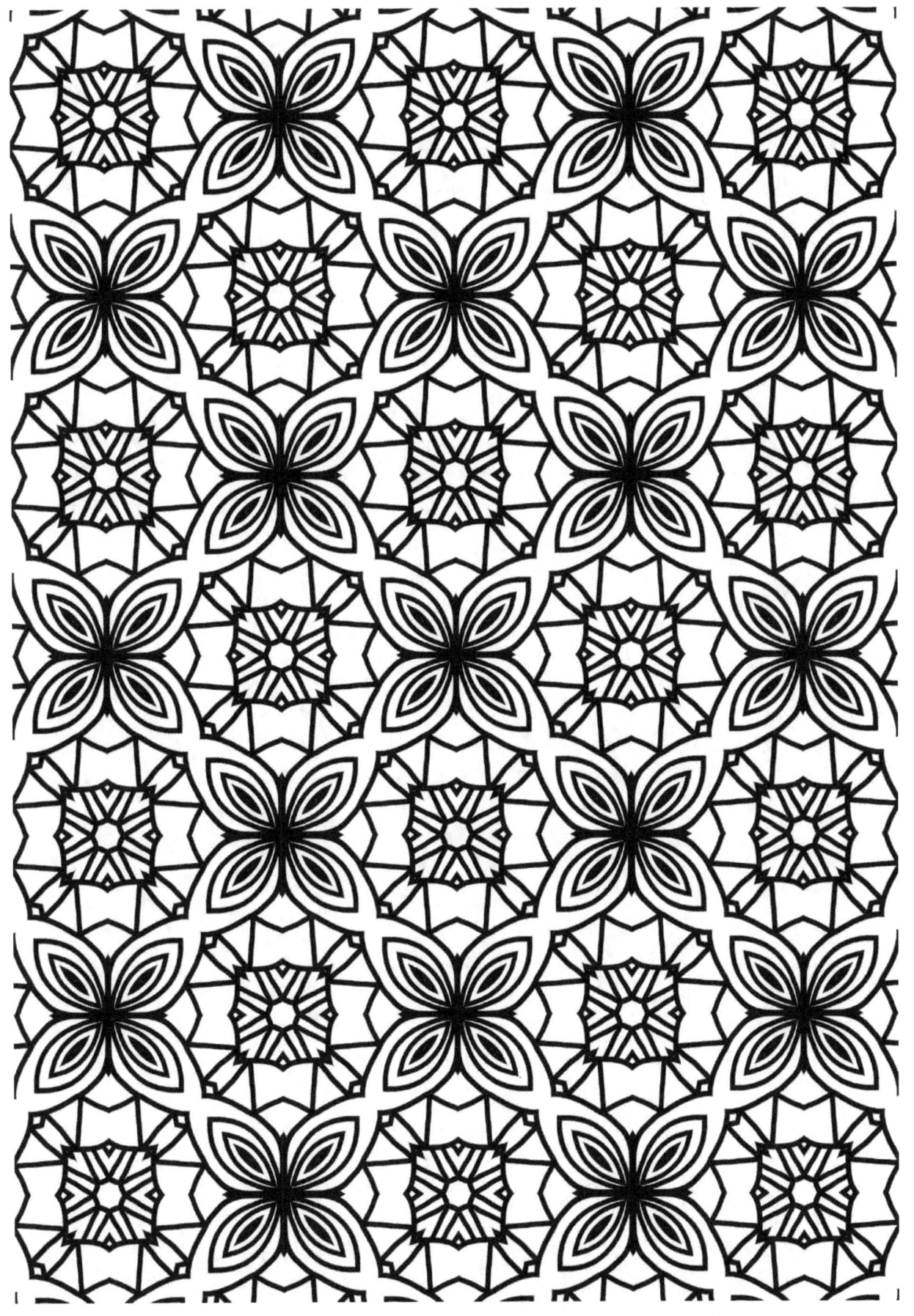

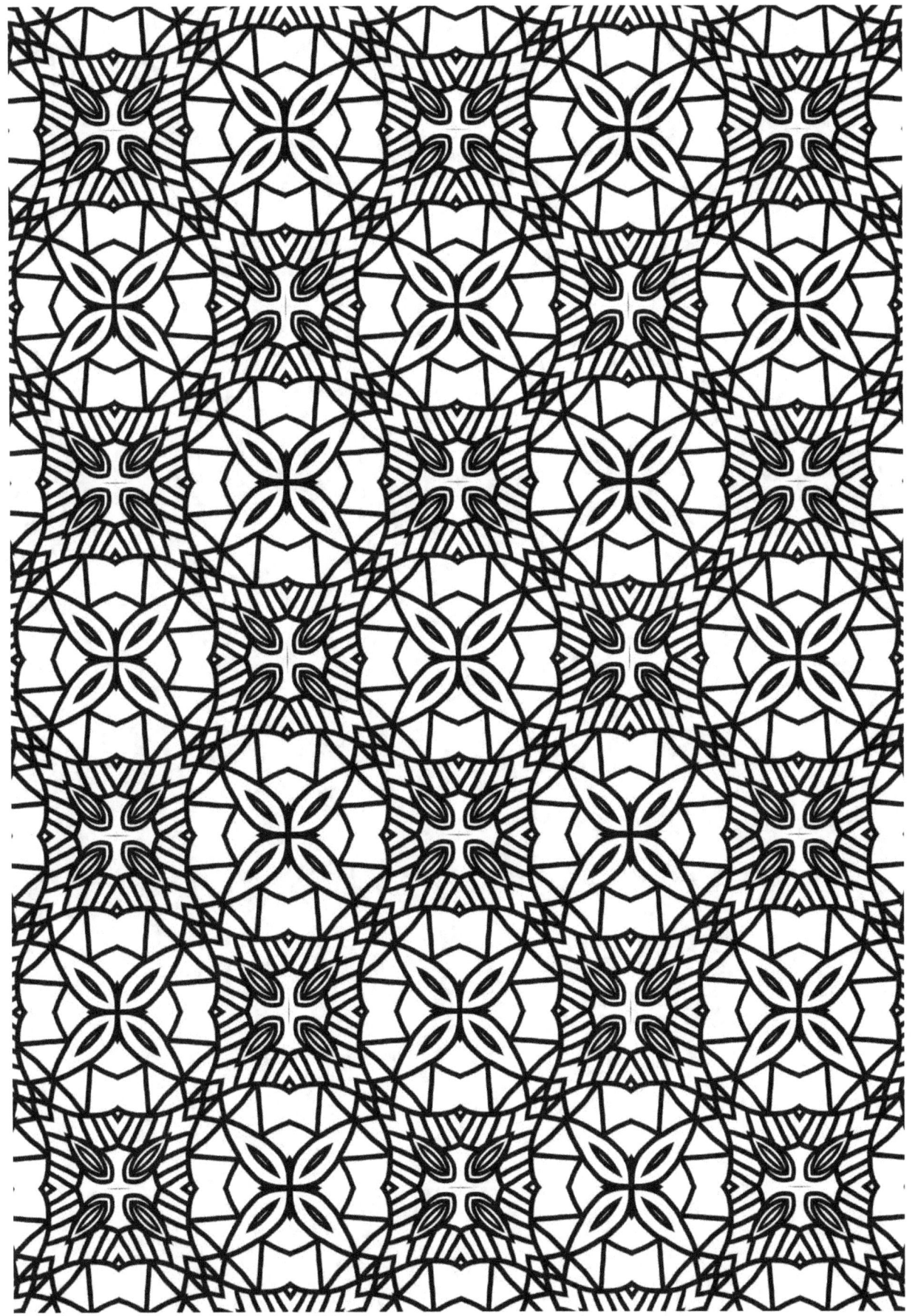

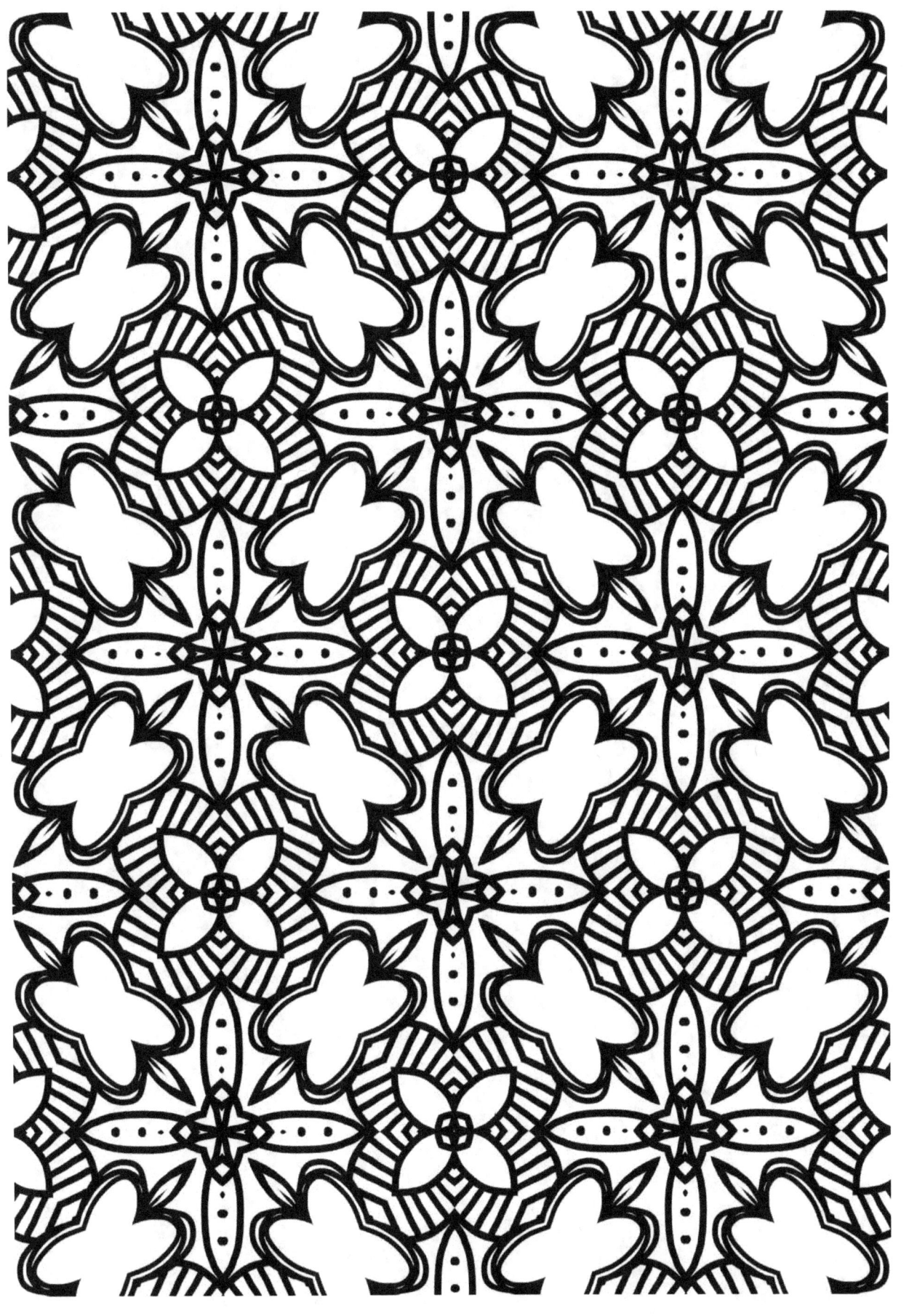

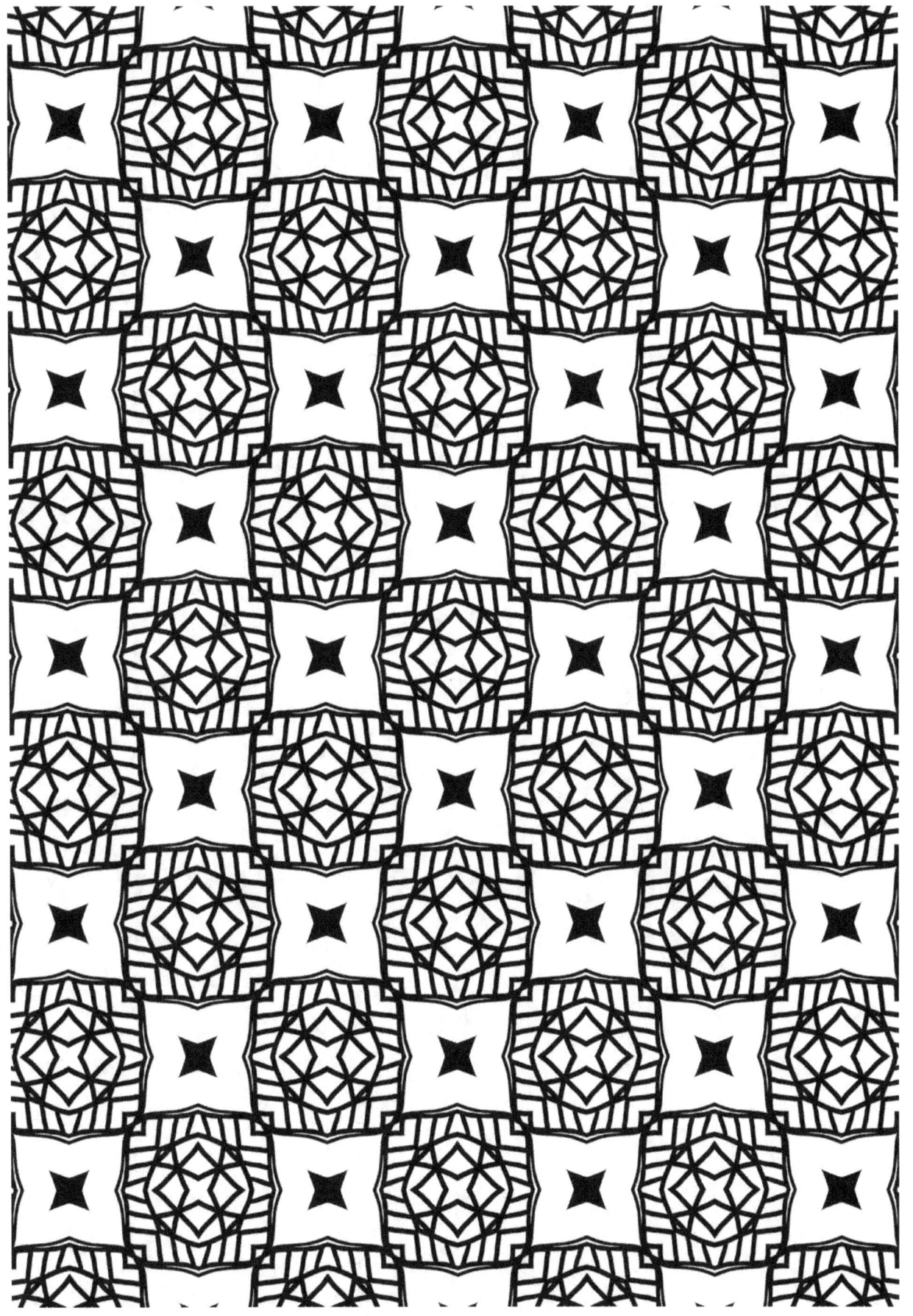

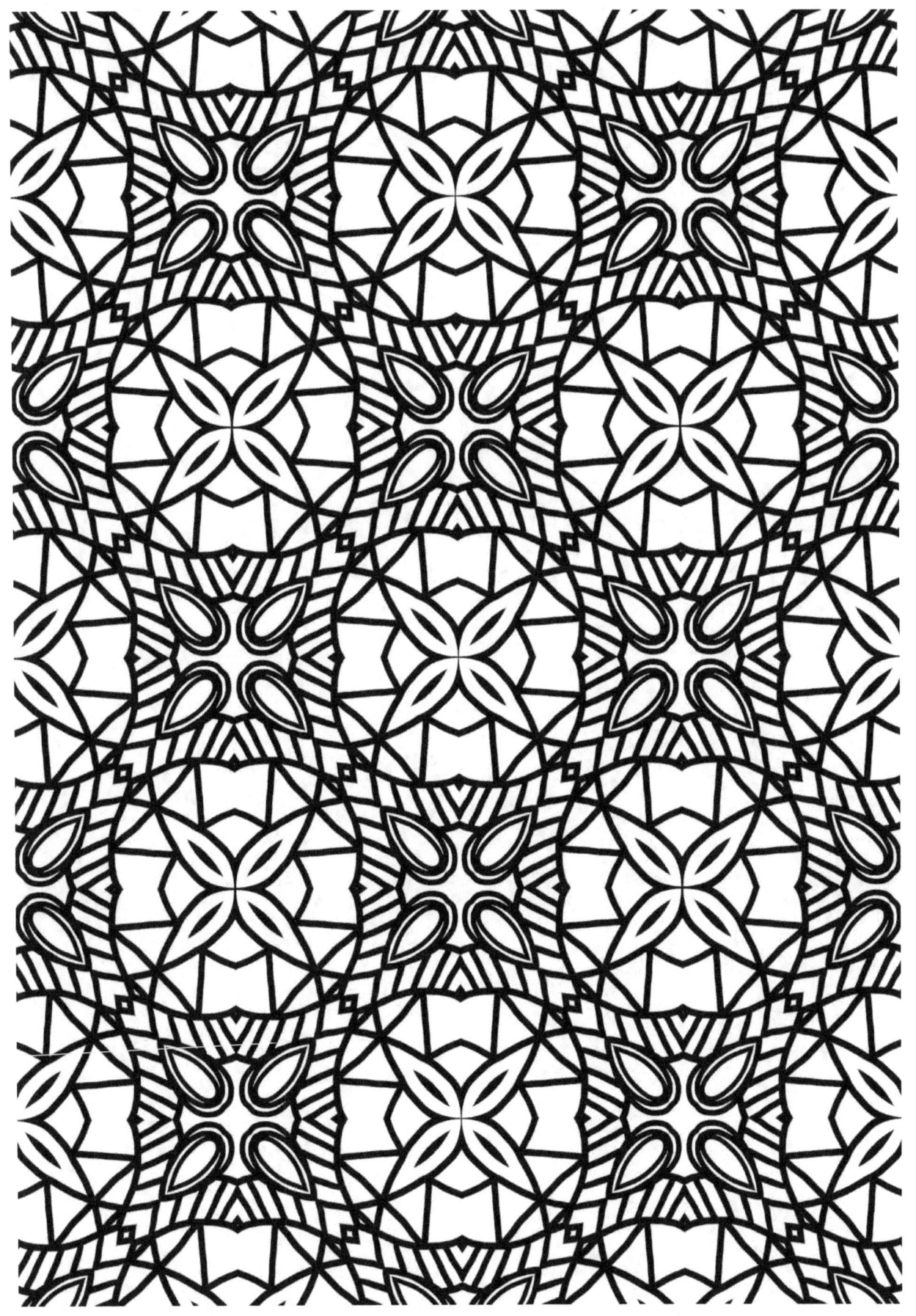

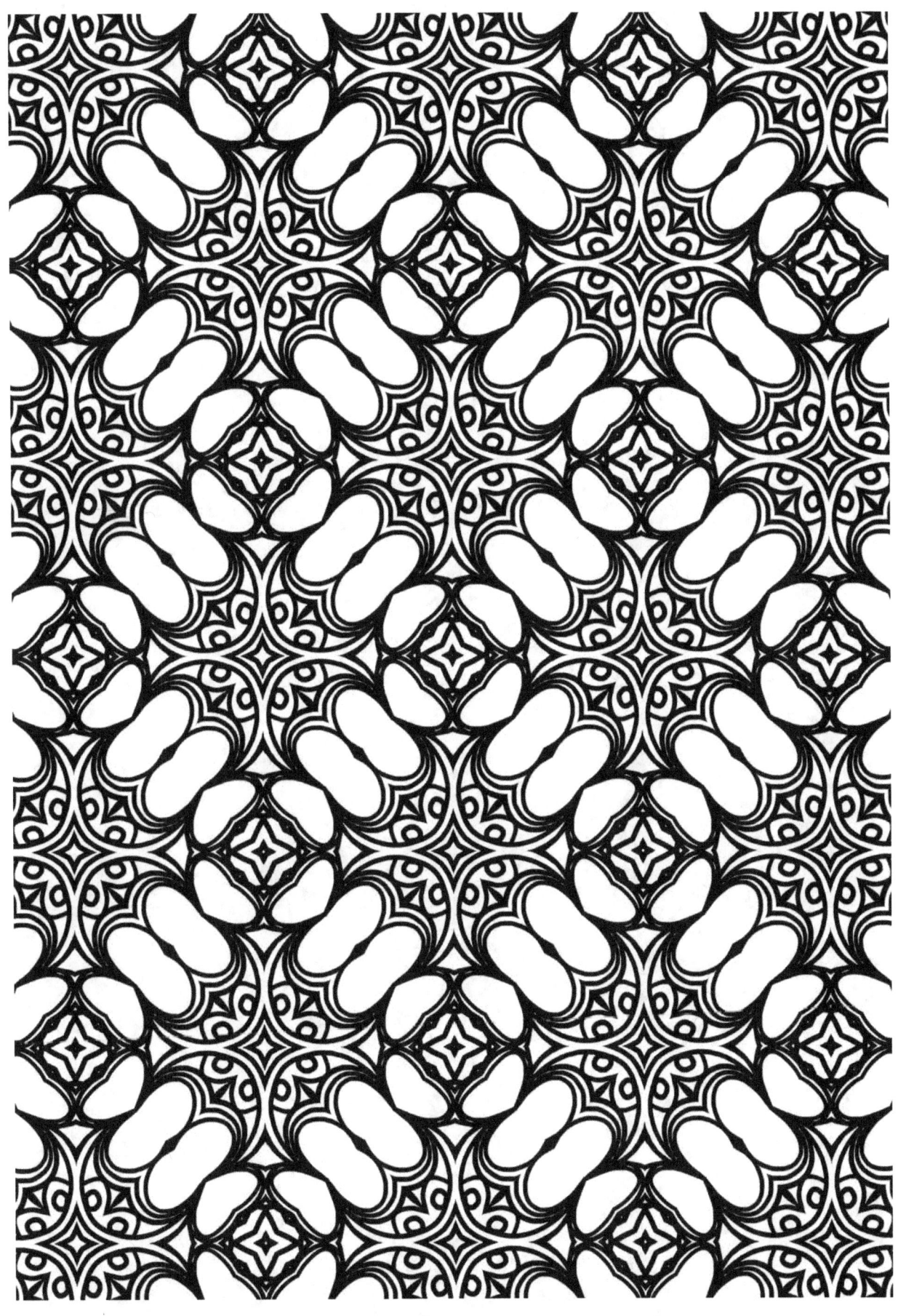

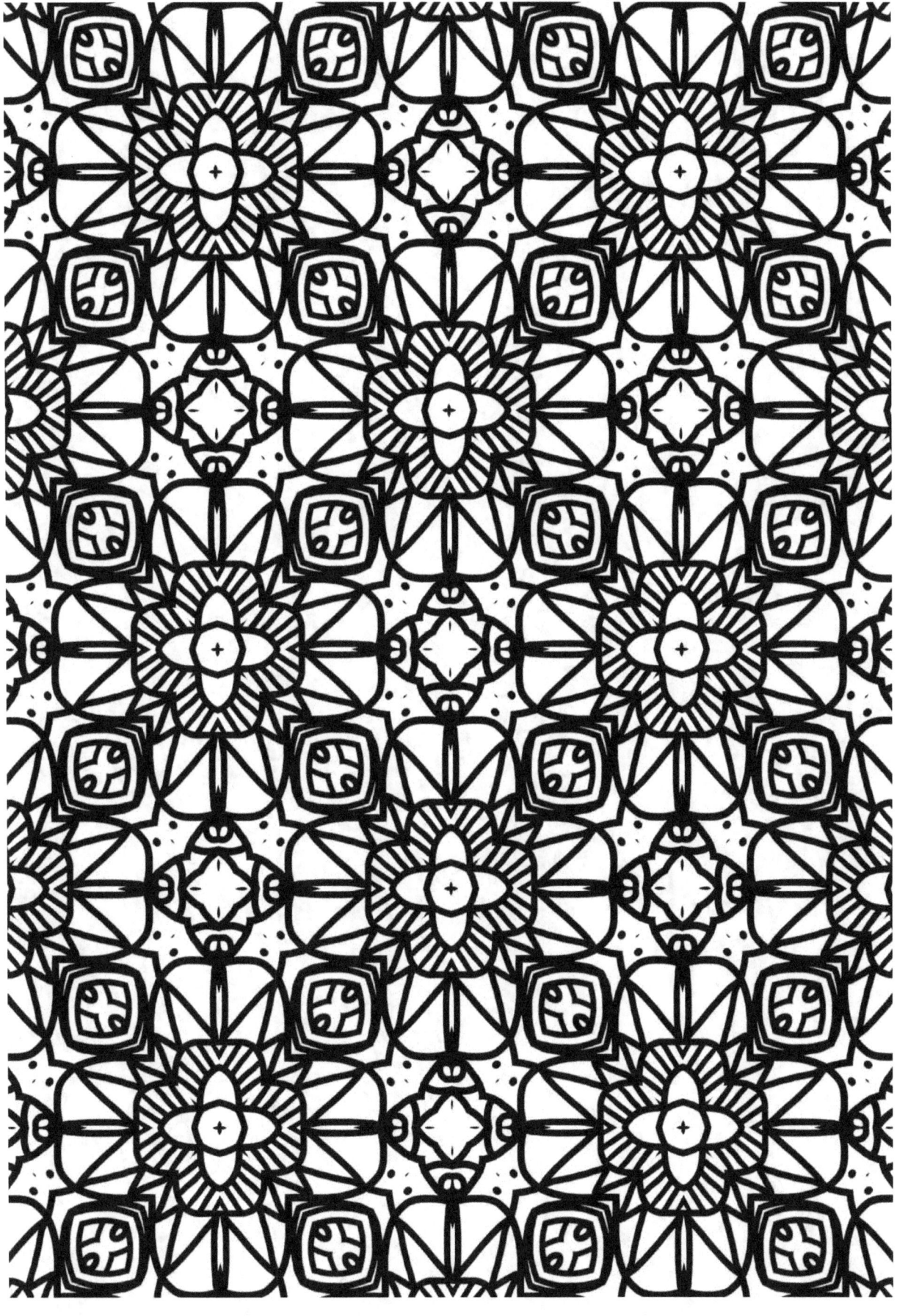

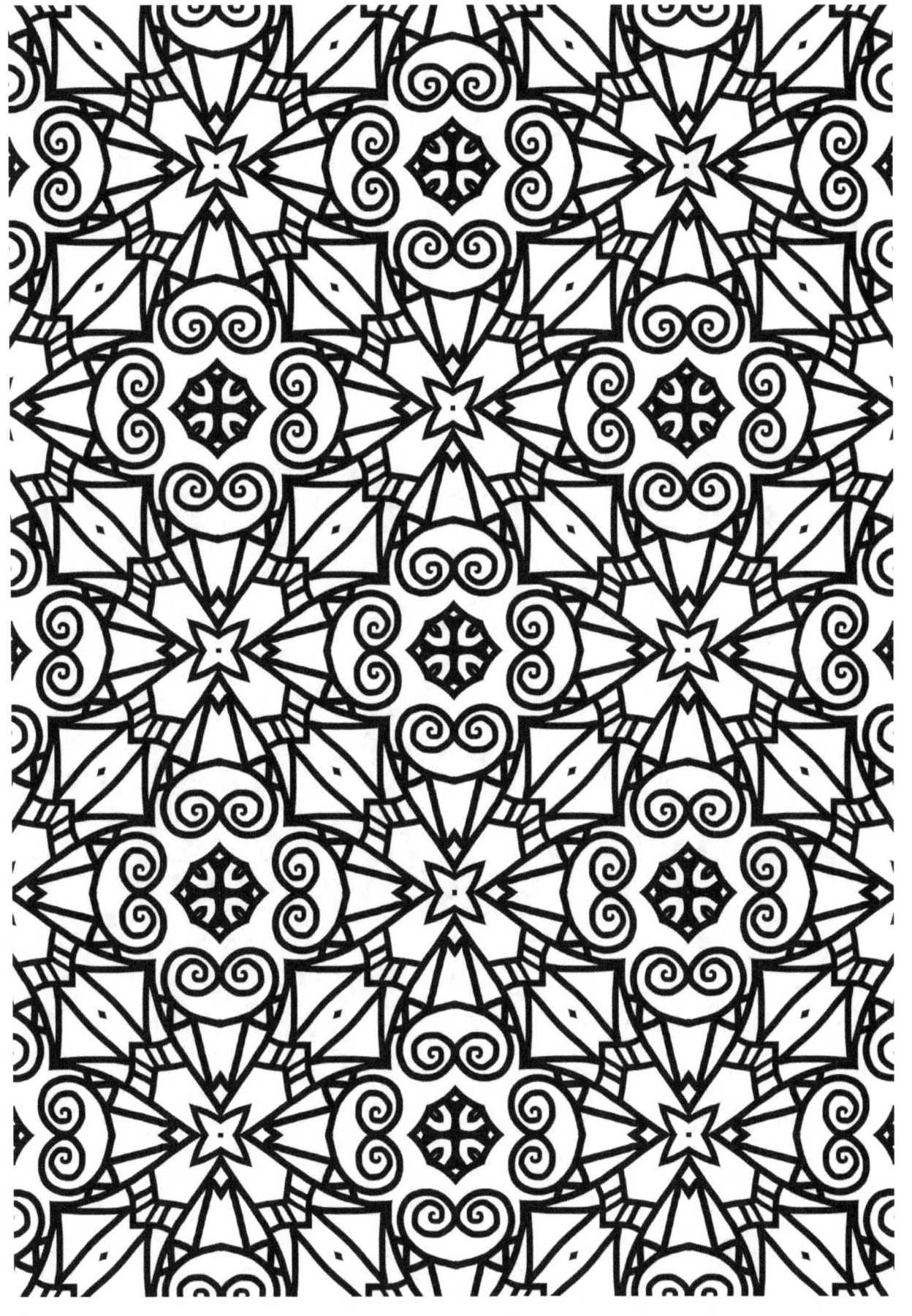

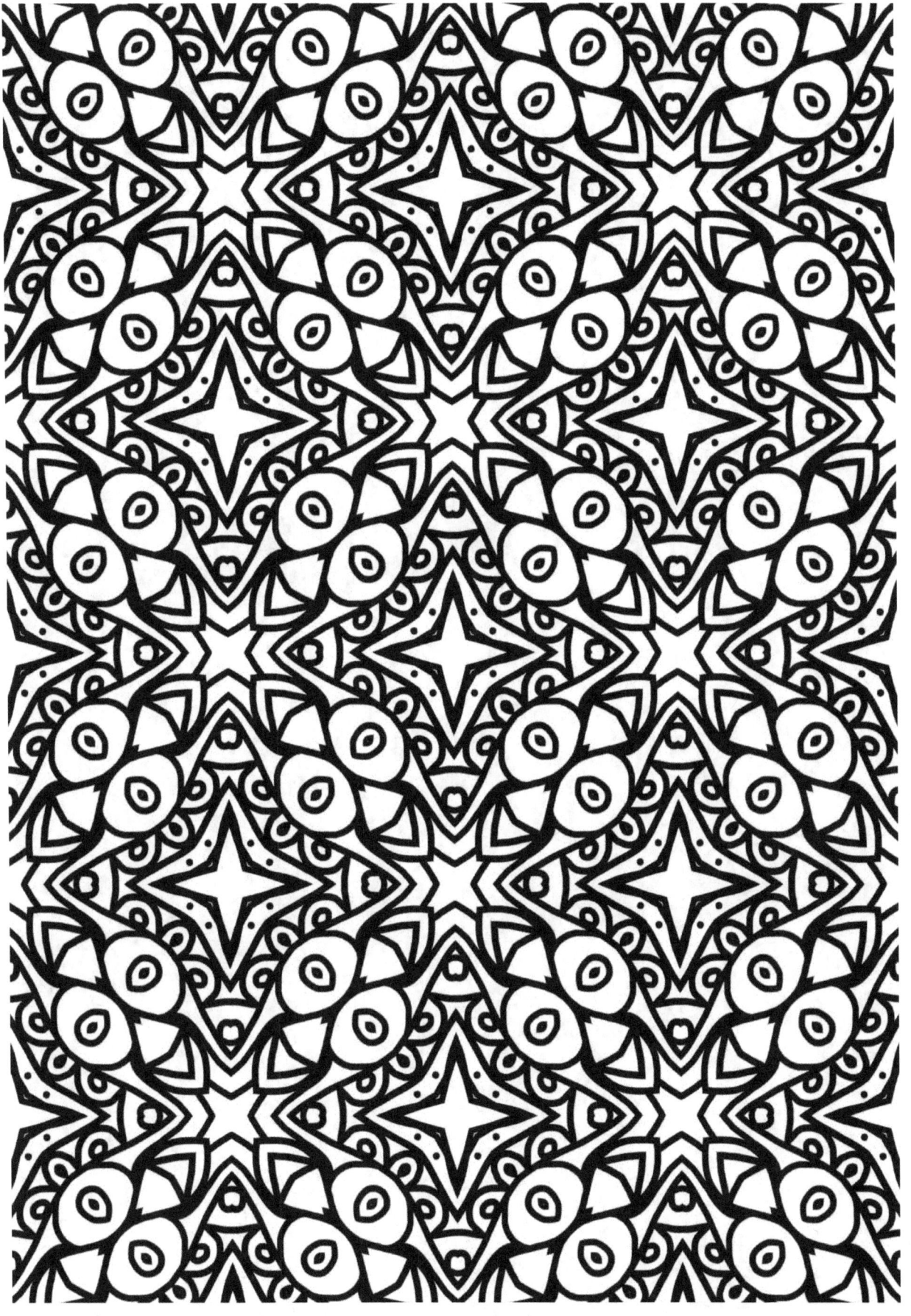

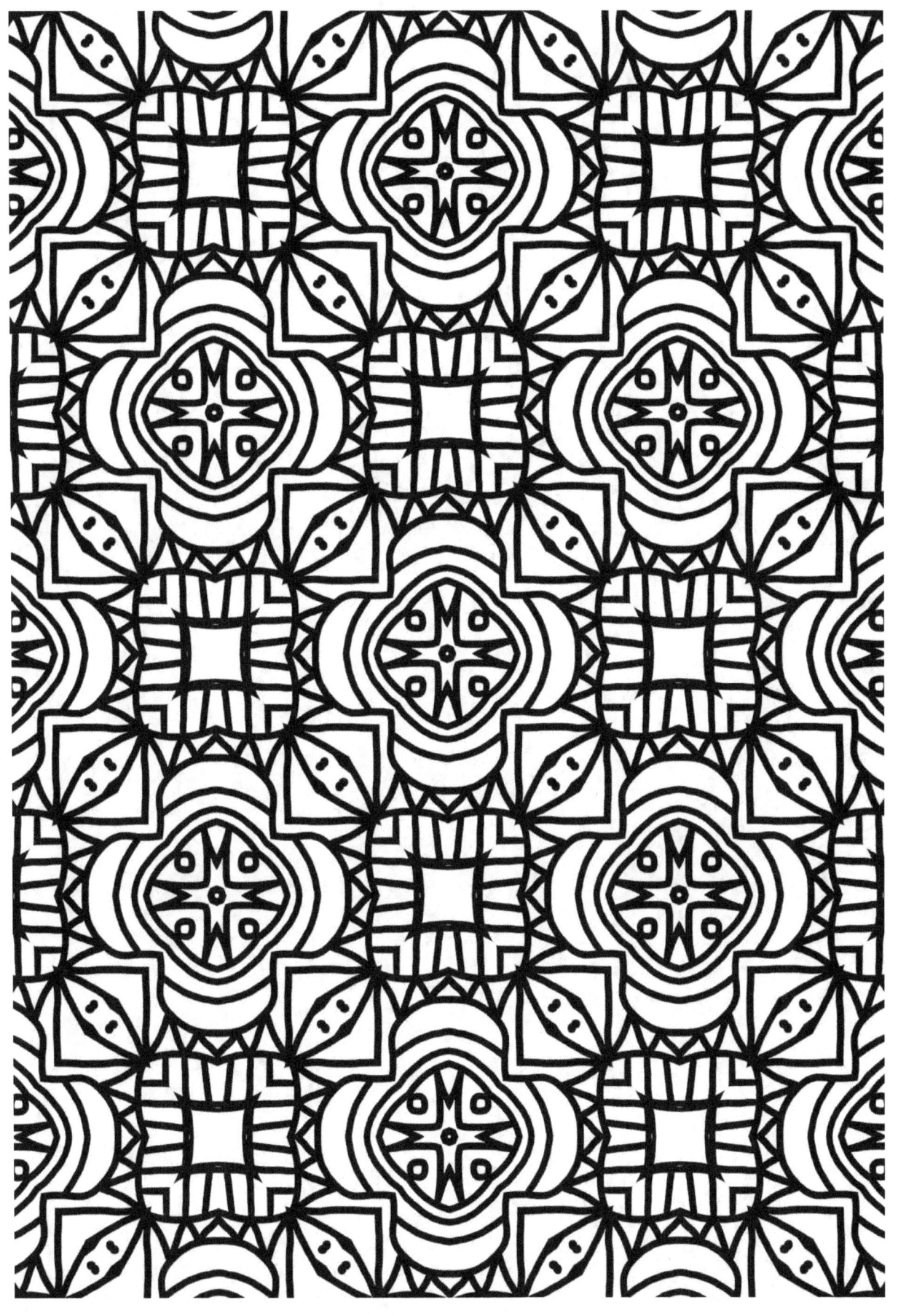

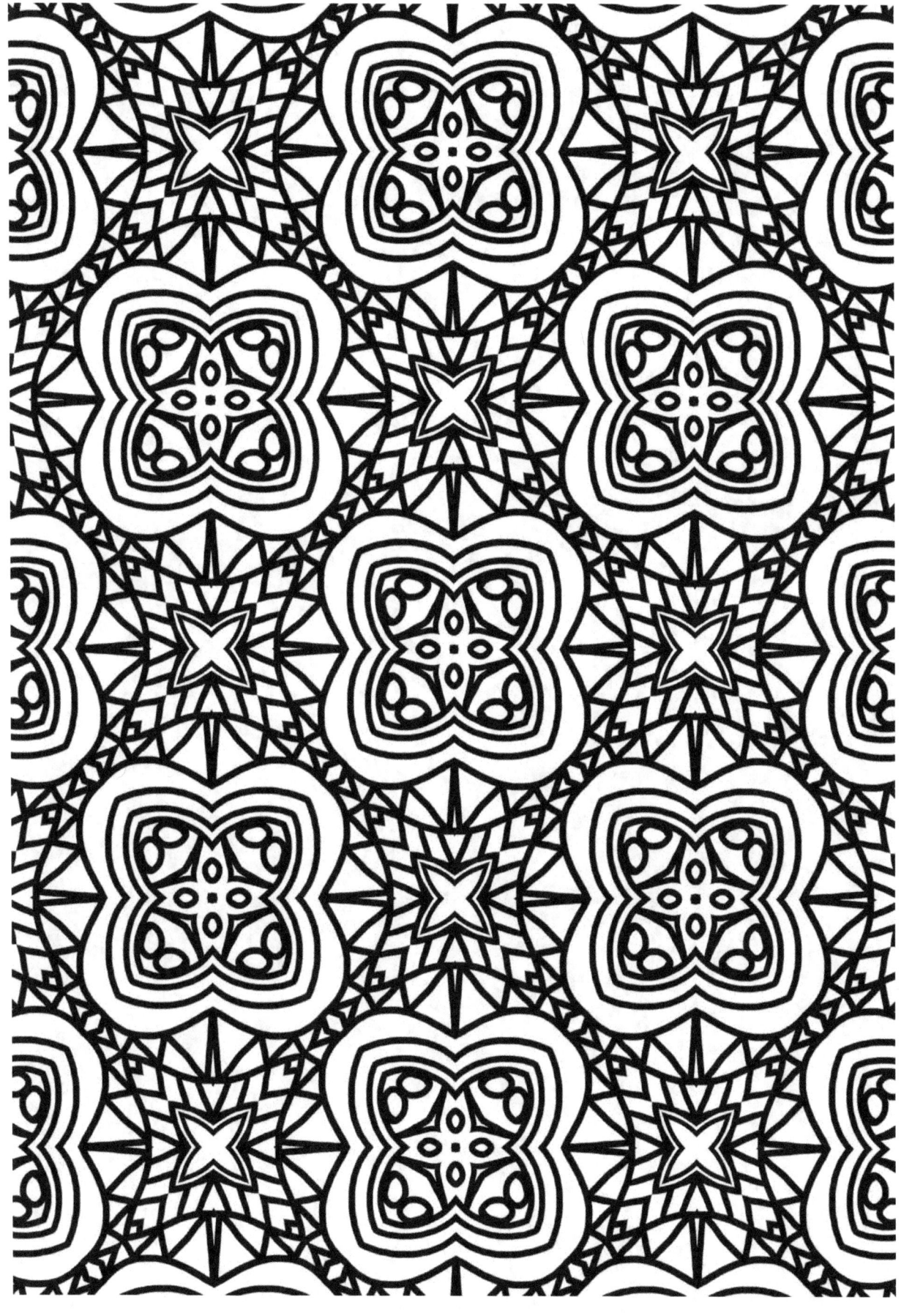

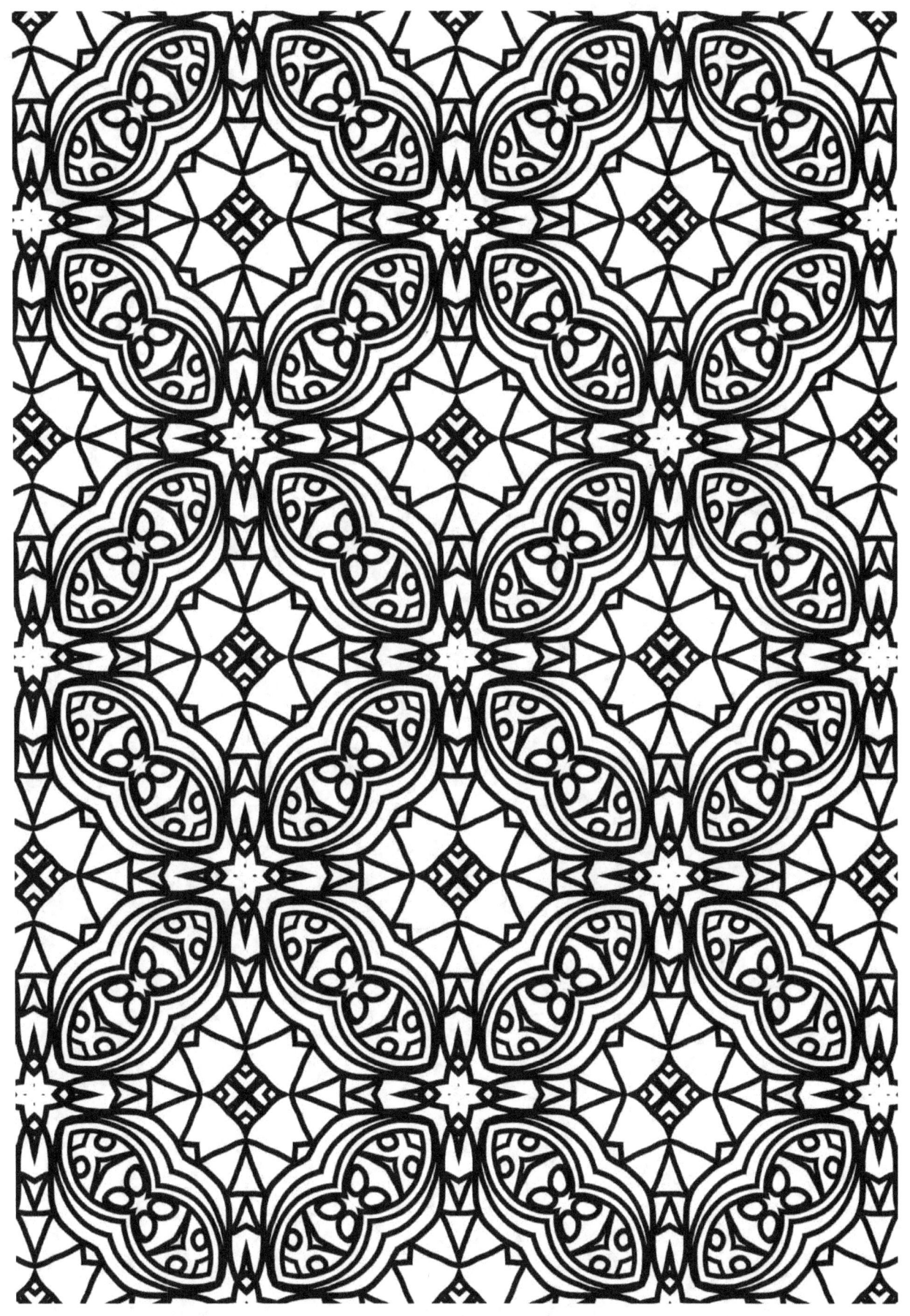

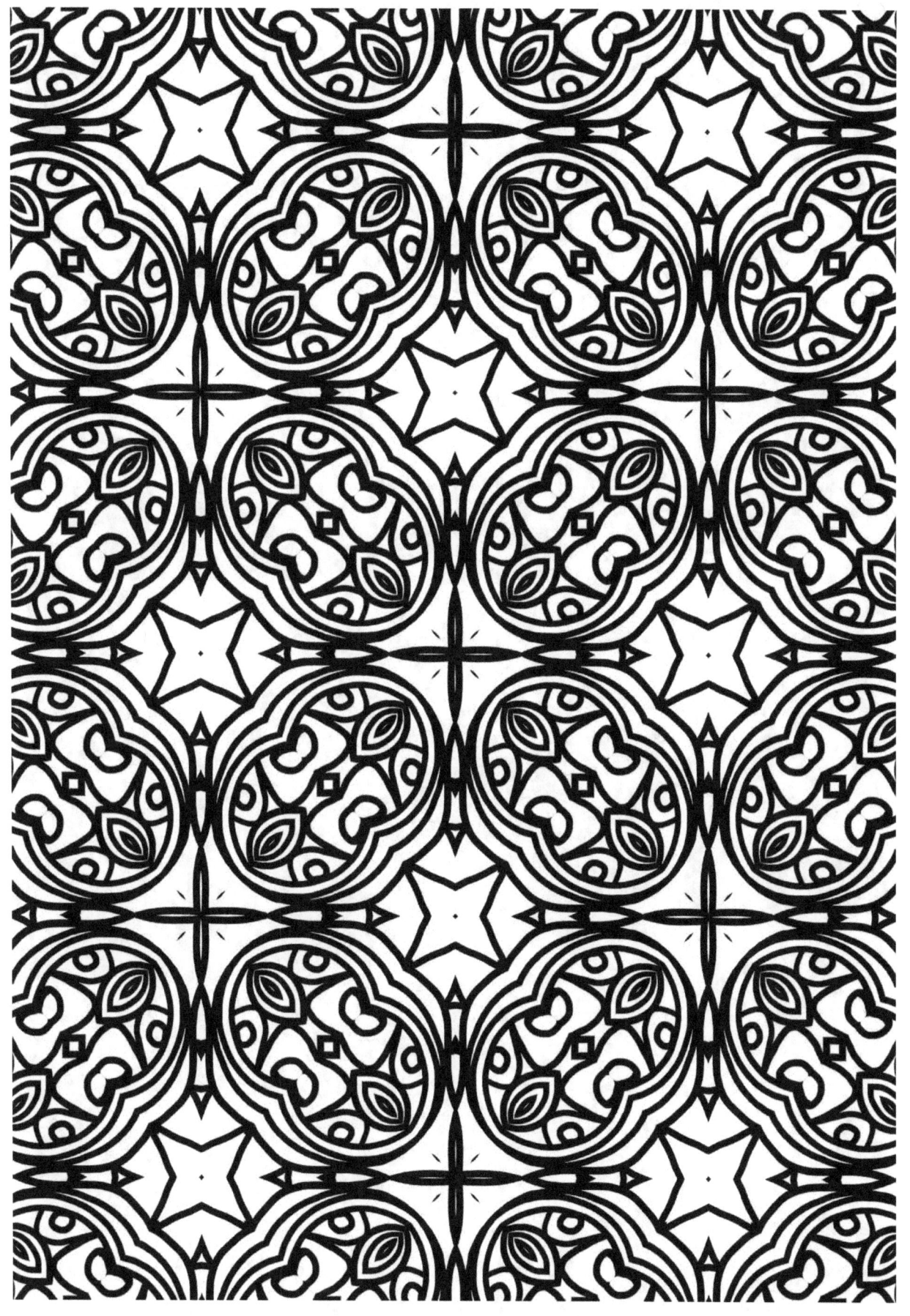

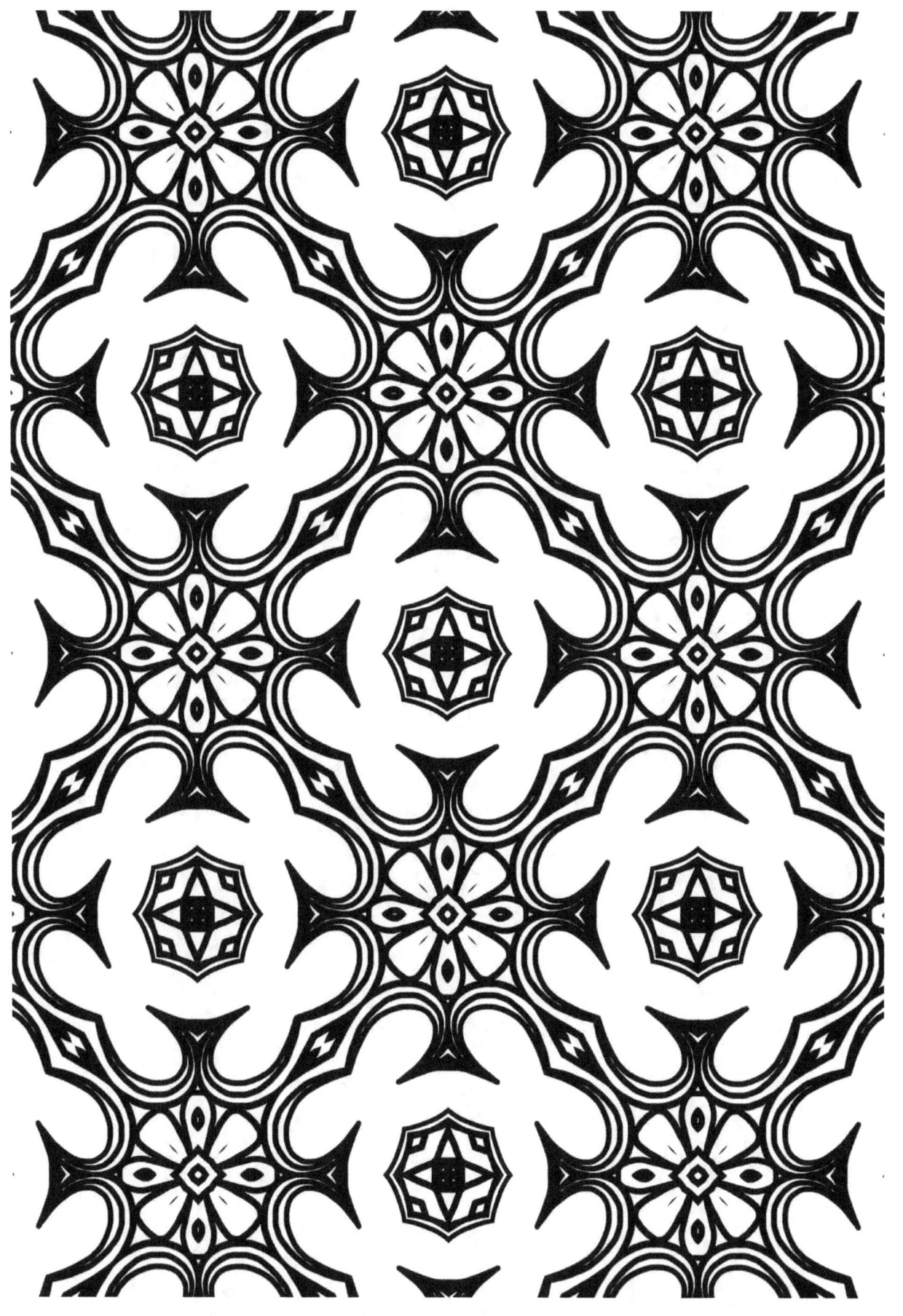

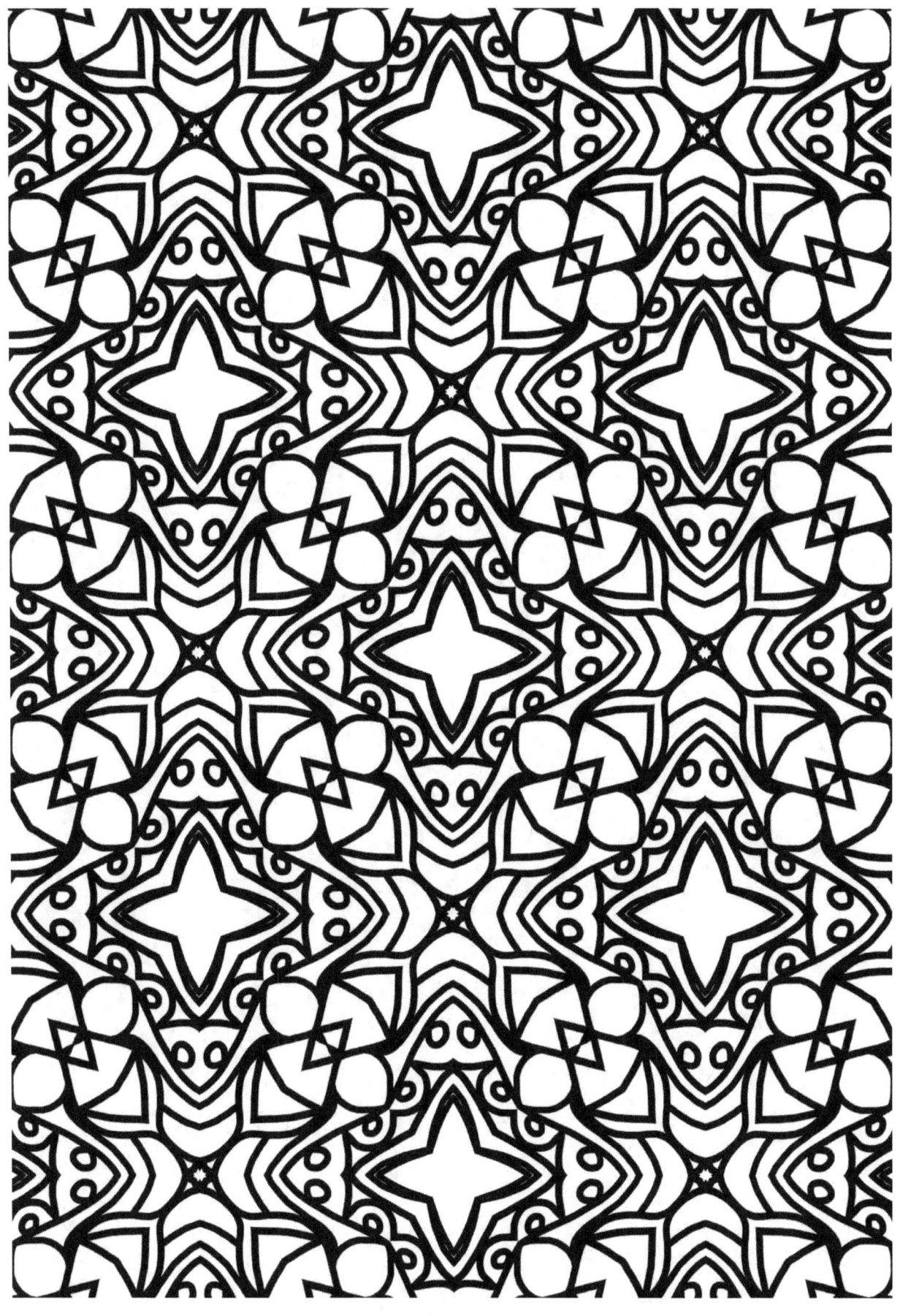

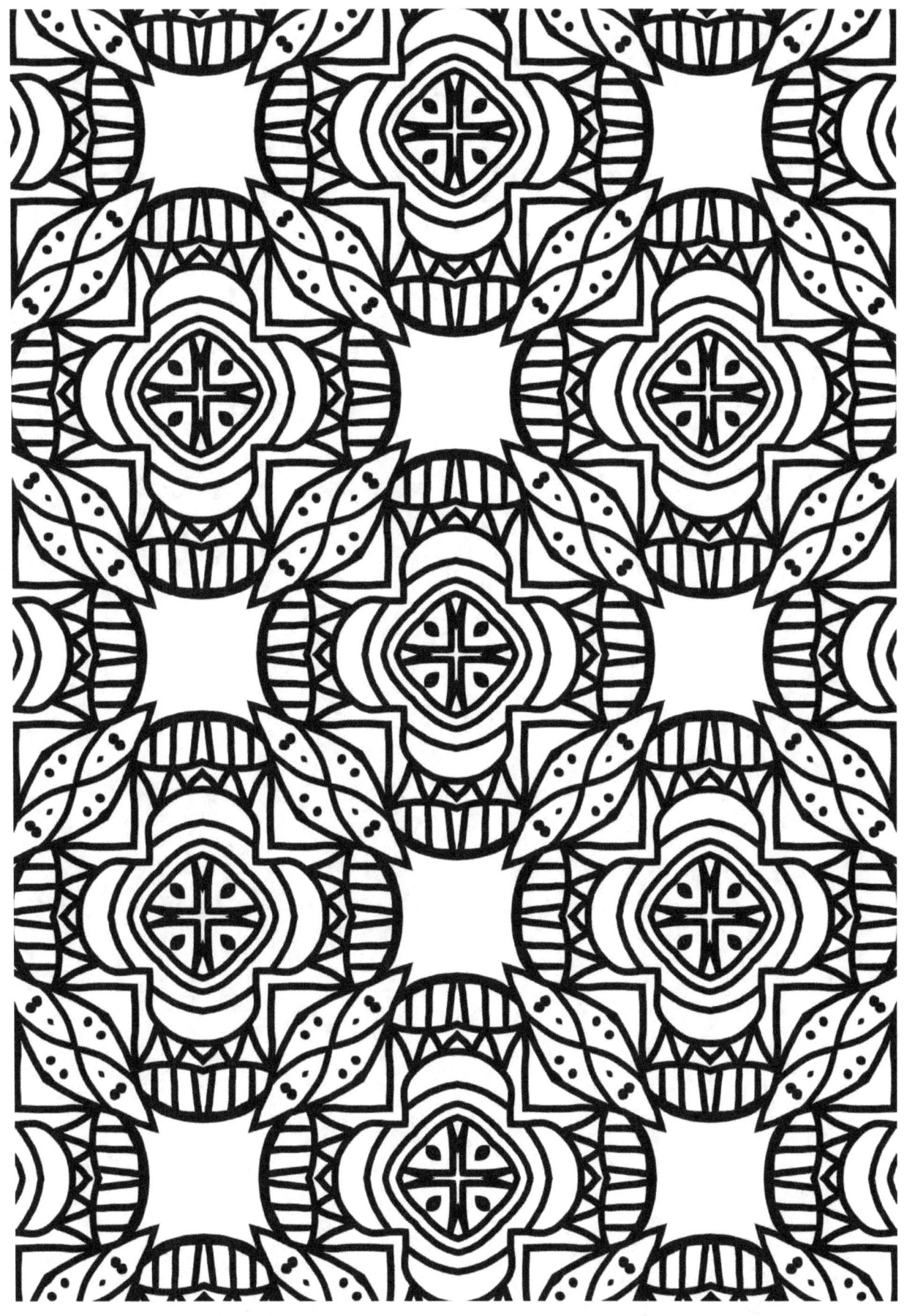

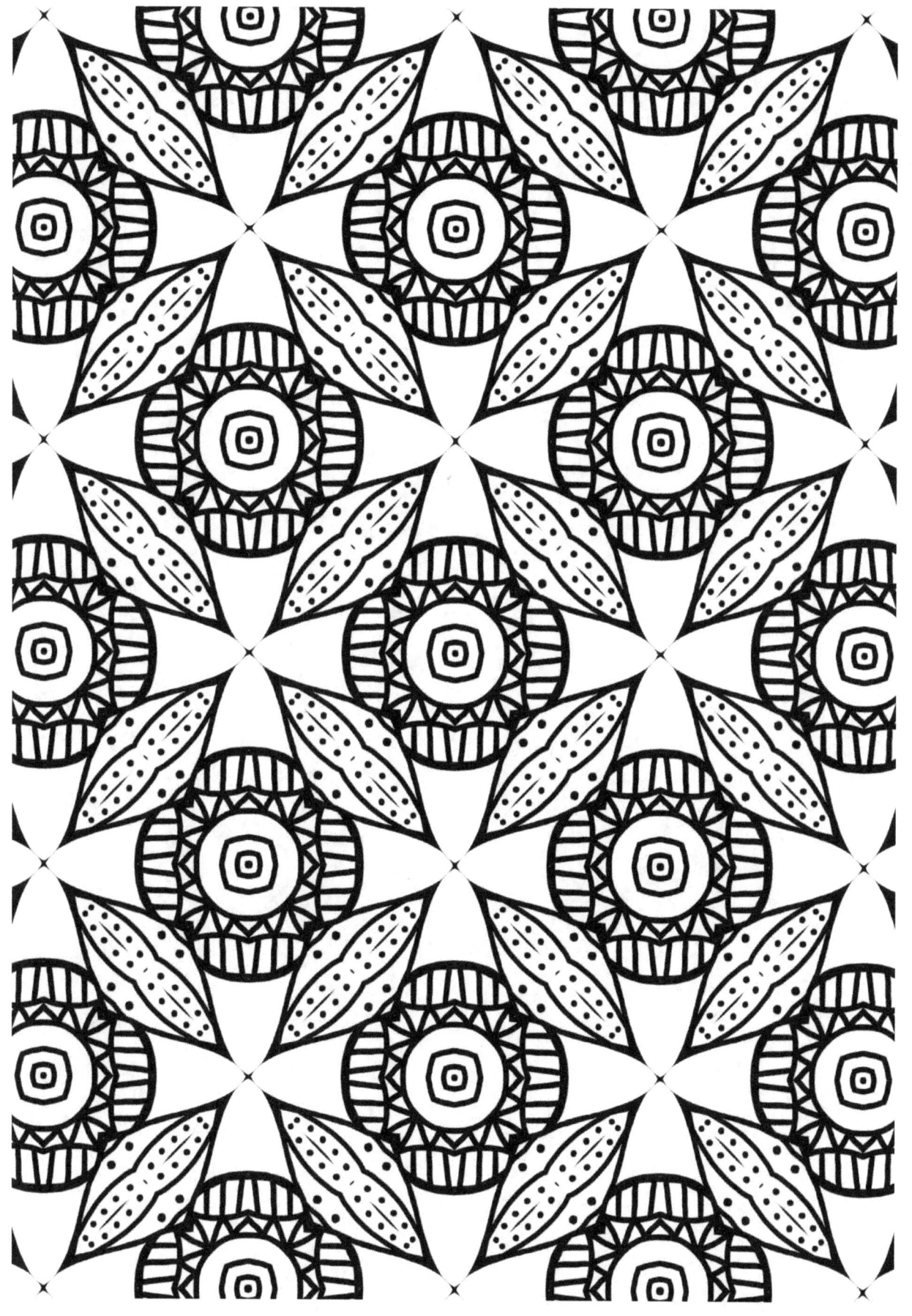

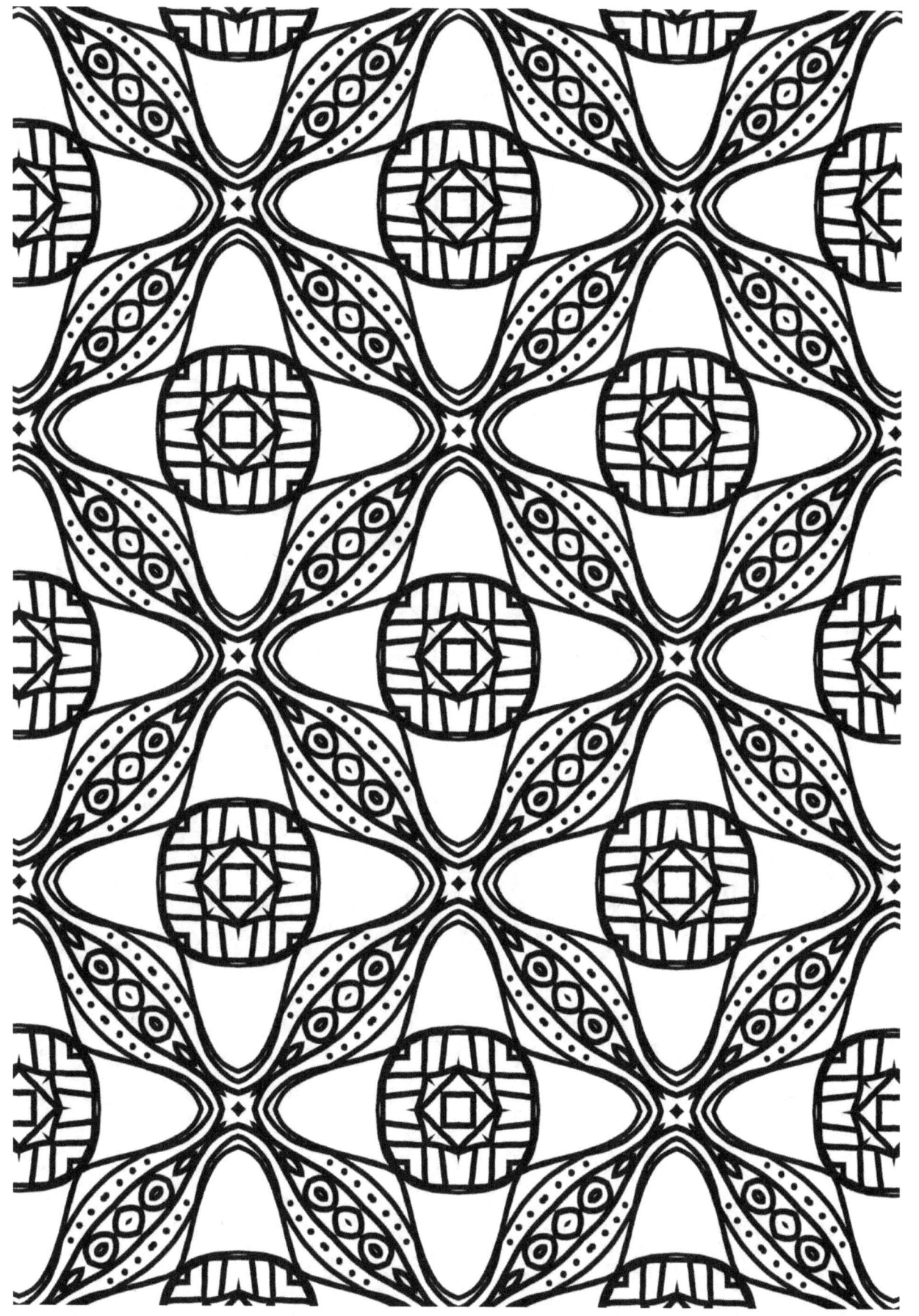

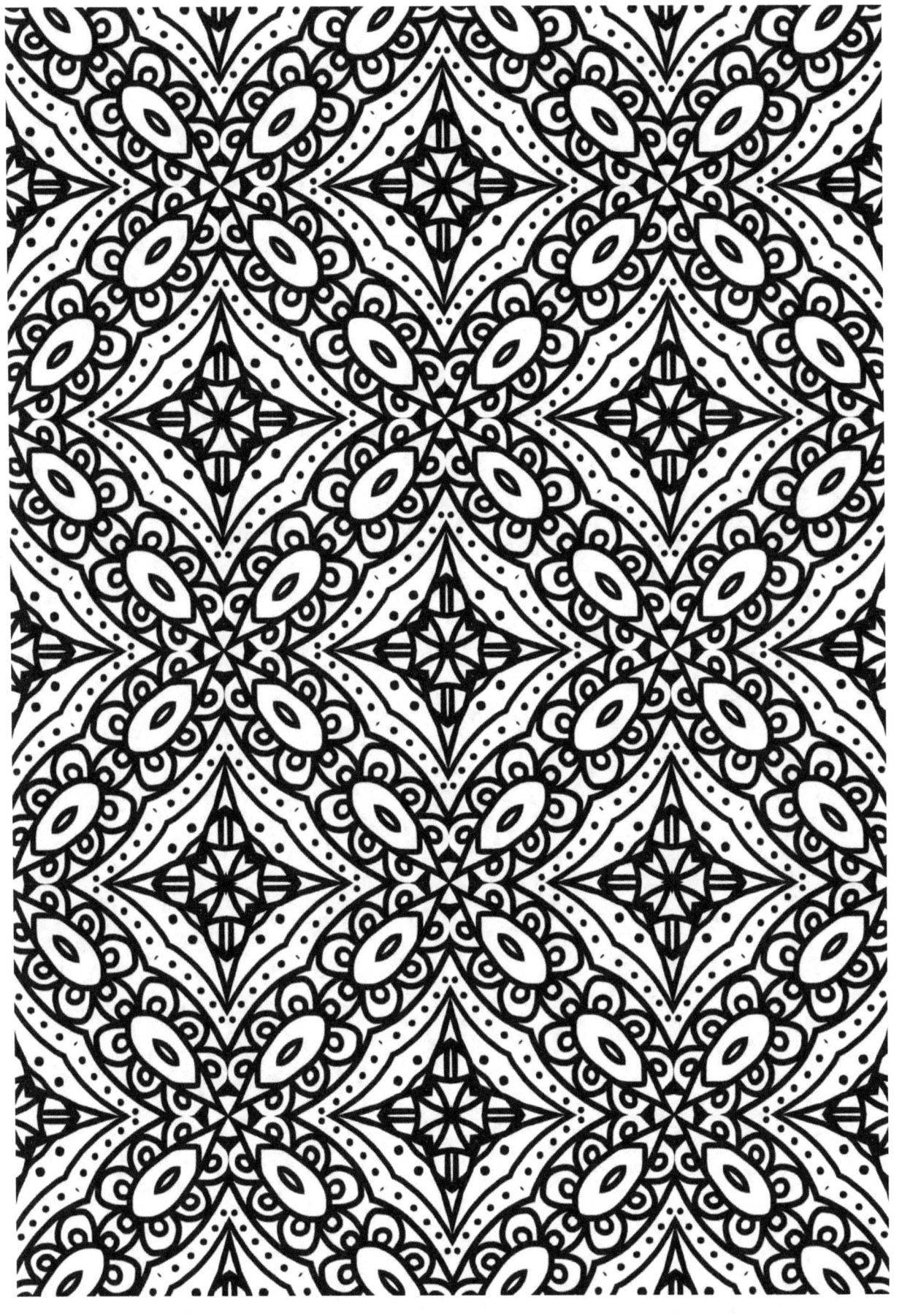

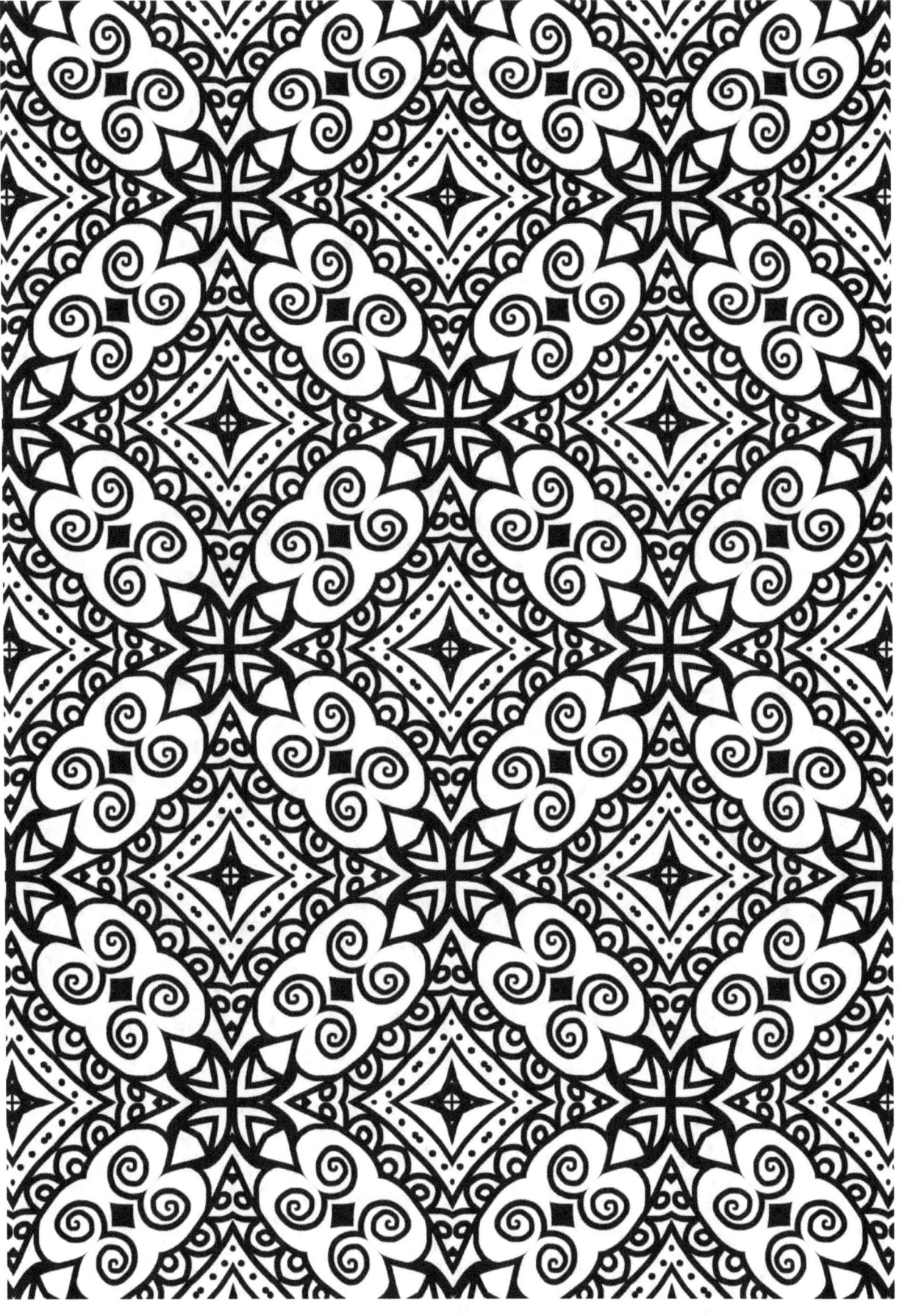

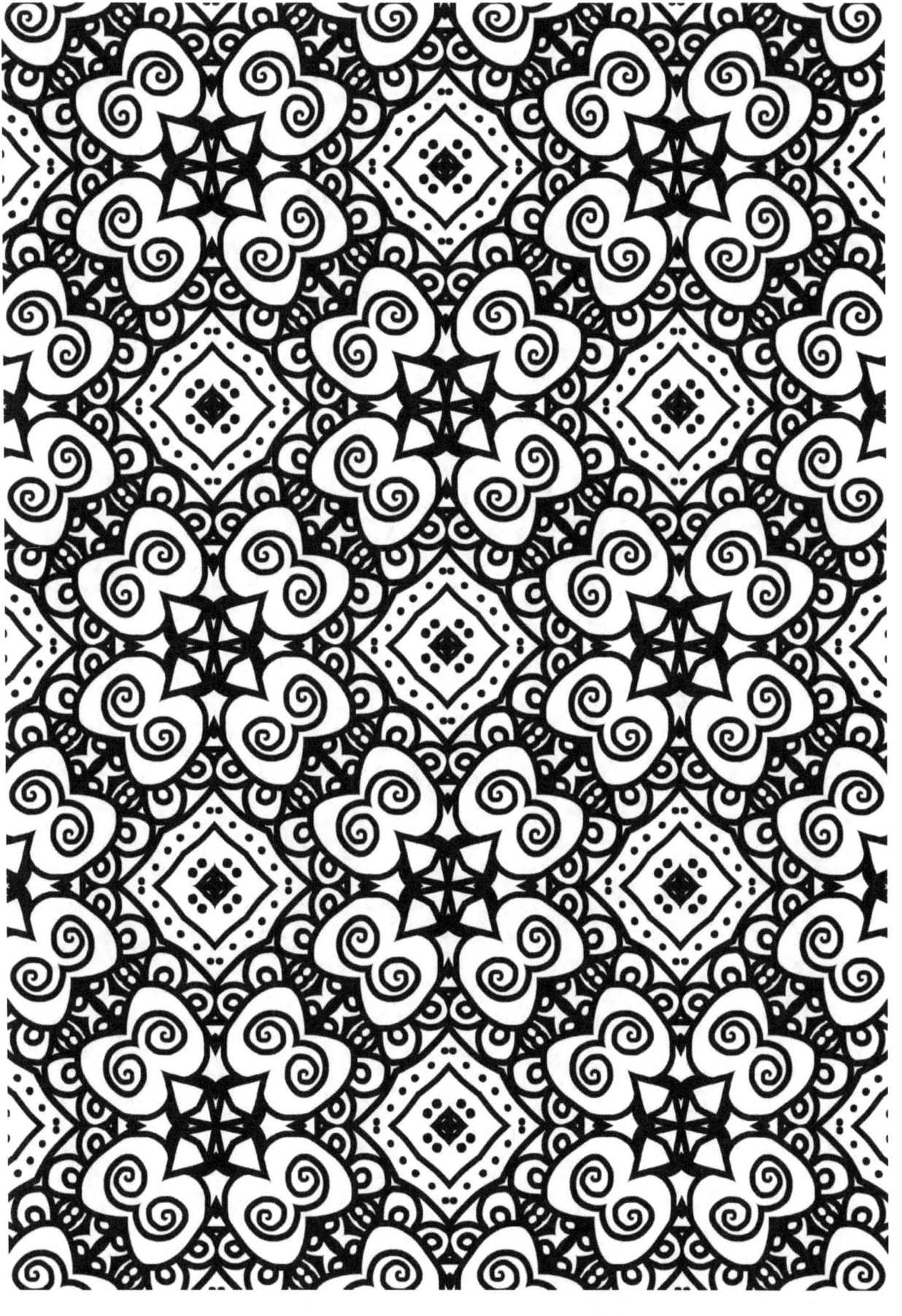

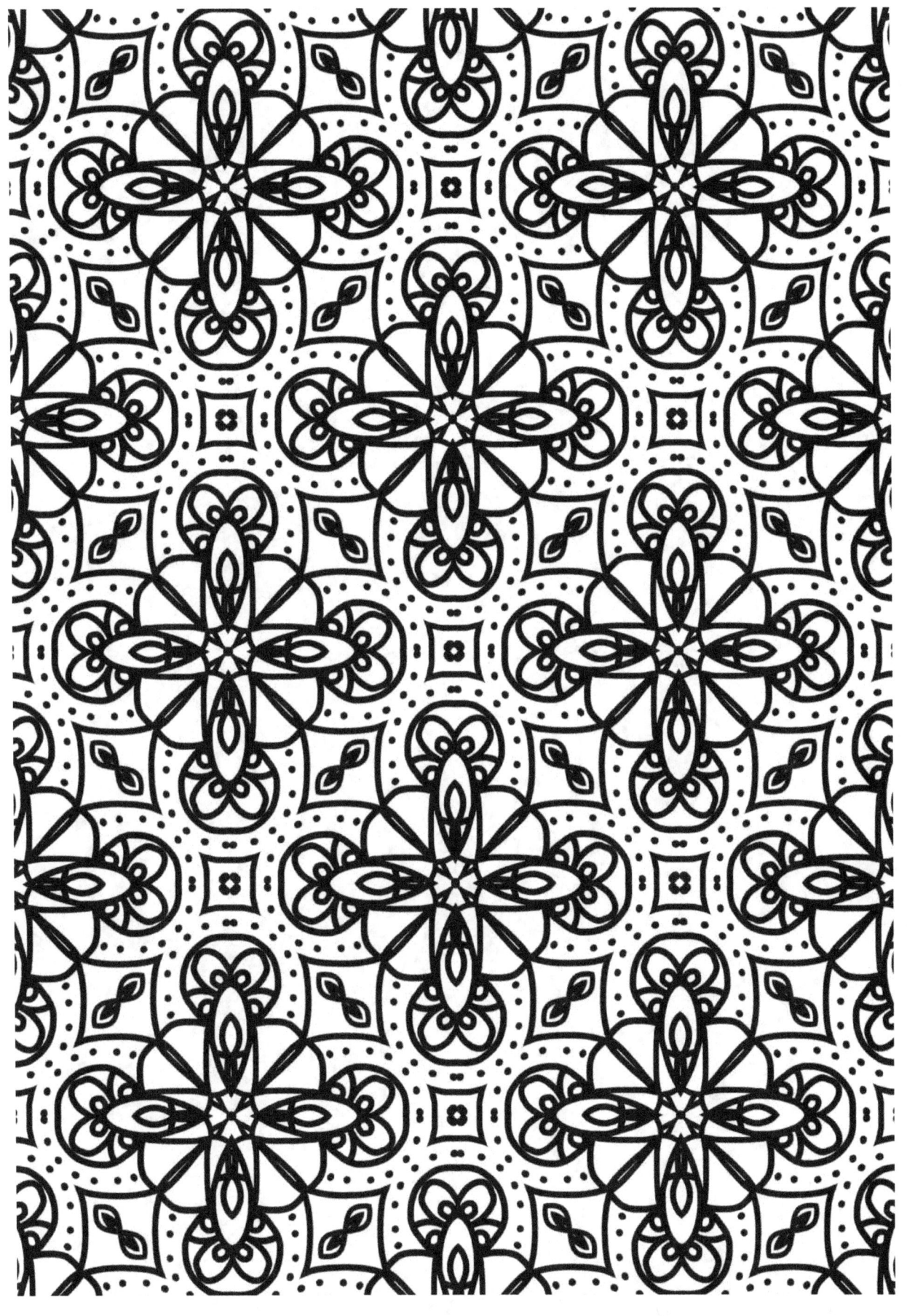

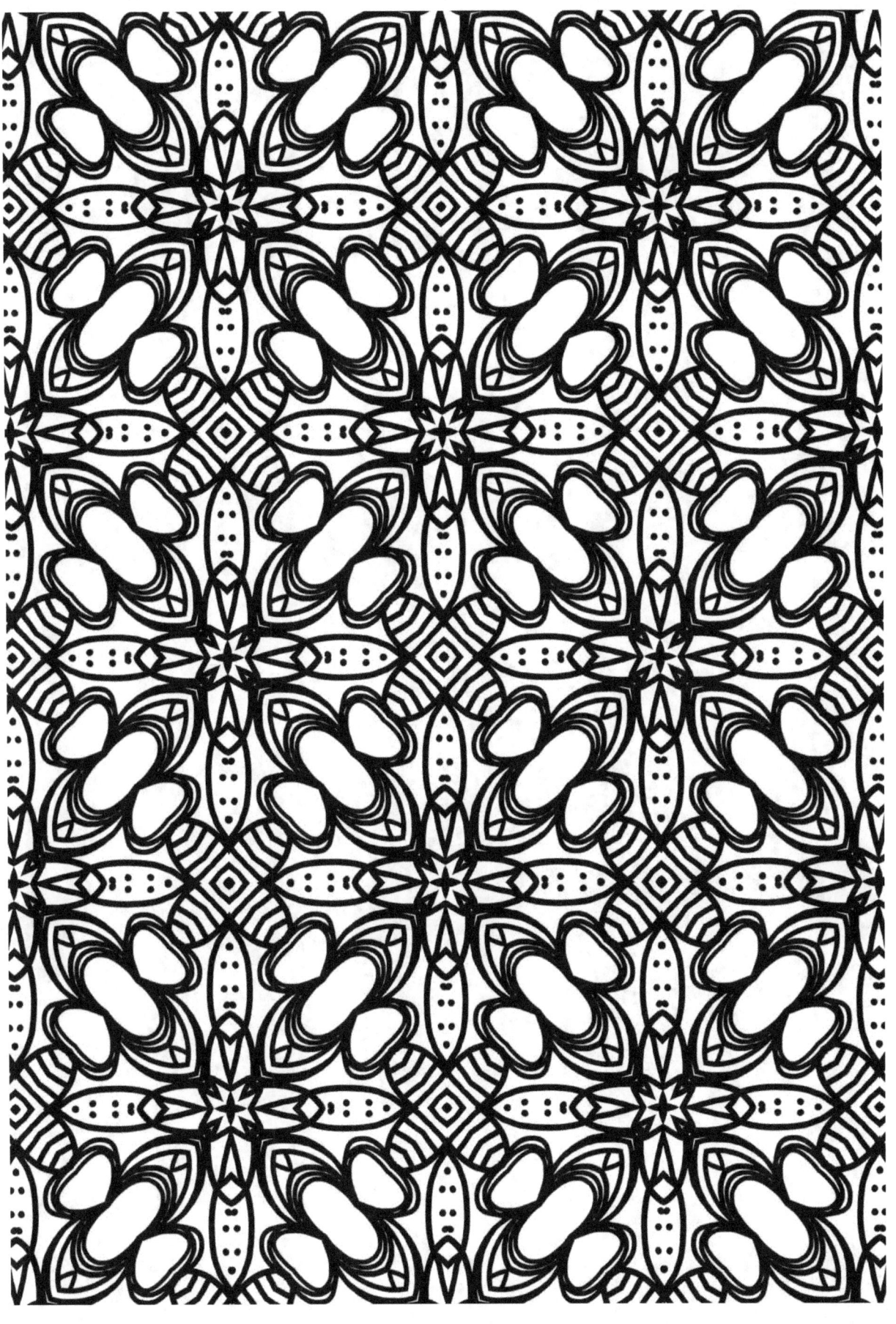

Conclusion

Congratulations! You become more relaxed and creative! In your life has become more colorful and fun! Prior to meeting with you in my new book **Adult Coloring Book 3** by **Maggie Dream.**